COMPUTATIONAL DRUG DISCOVERY

Prof Mohammed
Assistant Professor,
Department of Bioinformatics
Oxford Science College, Bangalore

Dr Shaik Jameel
Assistant Professor,
Department of Biotechnology
VIT University, Vellore

Author Message:

PUBLISHING FOR ONE WORLD

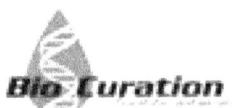

Biocuration infolabs
Jayanagar 1st Block
Bangalore-560011
Ph: +91 080-26560388, M: +91 -8553794025
Visit us at **www.biocurationssl.com**

Author Information

Prof Mohammed - Bioinformatician : He has 5 year of experience in Bioinformatics Research Industry along with his Research He participated in Visiting Faculty in various colleges for Bioinformatics Subjects.He is a Research fellow from **NCBS(TIFR), IISc, VIT UNIVERSITY**.He received DBT Fellowship and TATA GRANT Fellowship for his Research work. He has four publications in Bioinformatics tools Development.

PREFACE

This book has originated from Practical class on Genomics & Proteomics that are offered to students of Computational Biology, Bangalore University of Bangalore. The idea to write a book on Computational Biology was born during the preparations of these practical where I realized that it is extremely difficult to achieve an overview of the area of Drug Discovery and to follow the progress of this field. This is the first book in 2015 and was written in English .Computational Biology is a major topic in modern medical, Life science and pharmacological research and is of central importance in the computational biology science. Accordingly, The enormous increase in data on Drug Designing has led me to leave out the practical on Computational Biology and. This topic has since evolved into a huge research area of its own that could not be considered adequately within this book. My knowledge of Drug Designing practical has exploded in the past 5 years, Bioinformatics could be treated here with the same thoroughness. It is the aim of the present book to describe the Bioinformatics practical approach for life science students.

CONTENTS

COMPUTATIONAL DRUG DISCOVERY PROCESS

Introduction

Computational methods helped medication revelation/outline routines have assumed a noteworthy part in the improvement of restoratively vital little particles for more than three decades. These strategies are extensively named either structure-based or ligand-based techniques. Structure-based strategies are on a basic level similar to high-throughput screening in that both target and ligand structure data is basic. Structure-based methodologies incorporate ligand docking, pharmacophore, and ligand plan techniques. The article talks about hypothesis behind the most vital routines and late effective applications. Ligand-based routines utilize just ligand data for anticipating movement relying upon its comparability/uniqueness to beforehand known dynamic ligands. We audit generally utilized ligand-based routines, for example, ligand-based pharmacophores, atomic descriptors, and quantitative structure-action connections. Furthermore, essential apparatuses, for example, target/ligand information bases, homology demonstrating, ligand unique mark techniques, and so on., important for effective usage of different PC supported medication disclosure/outline systems in a medication revelation fight are examined. At last, computational techniques for harmfulness expectation and improvement for ideal physiologic properties are talked about with fruitful samples from writing.

Target Identification

Target distinguishing proof and approval is the first key stage in the drug-revelation pipeline (see Fig.1). By 2000, just around 500 medication targets had been accounted for (3, 4). The finish of human genome venture and various pathogen genomes discloses that there are 30,000 to 40,000 qualities and in any event the same number of proteins; a large number of these proteins are potential focuses for medication revelation. Be that as it may, distinguishing proof and approval of druggable focuses from a large number of applicant macromolecules is still a testing errand (5). Various advances for recognizing targets have been created as of late. Trial methodologies, for example, genomic and proteomic strategies are the significant instruments for target recognizable proof (6, 7). In any case, these routines have been demonstrated wasteful in target revelation on the grounds that they are arduous and tedious. What's more, it is to a great degree hard to get moderately clear data identified with medication focuses from colossal data created by genomics, declaration profiling, and proteomics (5). As complementarities to the exploratory systems, a progression of computational (in silico apparatuses have likewise been produced for target ID in late two decades (6, 8–12). When all is said in done, they can be ordered into succession based methodology also, structure-based methodology. Succession based methodology contributes to the courses of action of the target distinguishing proof by giving utilitarian data about target hopefuls and situating data to natural systems. Such routines incorporate grouping arrangement for quality determination, prioritization of protein families, quality and protein annotation, and interpretation information examination for microarray or quality chip. Here, we just present an extraordinary structure-based system for target identification reverse docking. Atomic docking has been a guaranteeing approach in lead revelation (2, 13) (likewise see dialog beneath). Converse docking.

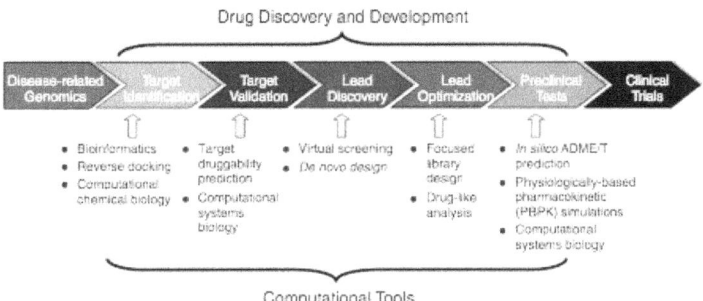

Figure 1 Computational approaches cover the drug-discovery pipeline, spanning from target identification to lead discovery to preclinical test.

In the fields of medicine, biotechnology and pharmacology, **drug discovery** is the process by which new candidate medications are discovered.

Verifiably, medications were found through recognizing the dynamic fixing from customary cures or by **serendipitous** disclosure. Later **chemical libraries** of manufactured small molecules, natural products or extracted were screened in place cells or entire living beings to recognize substances that have an alluring restorative impact in a procedure known as established pharmacology. Since sequencing of the human genome which permitted quick cloning and union of substantial amounts of refined proteins, it has gotten to be regular practice to utilize high throughput screening of expansive mixes libraries against separated biological targets which are estimated to be malady altering in a procedure known as reverse pharmacology. Hits from these screens are then tried in cells and after that in creatures for viability. Advanced medication revelation includes the identification of screening hits, Medical chemistry and streamlining of those hits to build the affinity, selectivity (to diminish the capability of reactions), viability/intensity, metabolic solidness (to expand the half-life), and oral bioavailability. When an intensify that satisfies these necessities has been distinguished, it will start the procedure of medication improvement preceding clinical trials. One or a greater amount of these steps might, yet not so much, include PC helped medication outline. Current medication revelation is subsequently generally a capital-serious procedure that includes substantial ventures by pharmaceutical industry organizations and also national governments (who give gives and credit ensures). In spite of advances in innovation and comprehension of natural frameworks, drug disclosure is still a protracted, "lavish, troublesome, and wasteful methodology" with low rate of new helpful revelation.

In 2010,the research and development cost of each new molecular entity was approximately US$ 1.8 billion. Drug disclosure is carried out by pharmaceutical organizations, with examination help from colleges. The "last item" of medication revelation is a patent on the potential medication. The medication requires extremely costly Phase I, II and III clinical trials, and the vast majority of them come up short. Little organizations have a basic part, regularly then offering the rights to bigger organizations that have the assets to run the clinical trials.

Finding medications that may be a business achievement, or a general wellbeing achievement, includes a complex collaboration between speculators, industry, the educated community, patent laws, administrative selectiveness, advertising and the need to adjust mystery with correspondence. In the mean time, for scatters whose irregularity implies that no huge business achievement or general wellbeing impact can be normal, the vagrant medication financing methodology guarantees that individuals who experience those issue can have some trust of pharmacotherapeutic advances.

Drug Targets

The meaning of "target" itself is something contended inside the pharmaceutical business. For the most part, the "target" is the characteristically existing cell or sub-atomic structure included in the pathology of investment that the medication being developed is intended to follow up on. On the other hand, the qualification between "another" and "created" target can be made without a full comprehension of simply what a "target" is. This qualification is normally made by pharmaceutical organizations occupied with revelation and advancement of therapeutics. In an appraisal from 2011, 435 human genome items were recognized as remedial medication focuses of FDA-affirmed medications

"Secured targets" are those for which there is a decent experimental understanding, supported by a long production history, of both how the target capacities in ordinary physiology and how it is included in human pathology. This does not suggest that the component of activity of medications that are thought to act through a specific built targets is completely caught on. Rather, "settled" relates straightforwardly to the measure of foundation data accessible on a focus, specifically practical data. The all the more such data is accessible, the less venture is (for the most part) needed to add to a remedial coordinated against the target. The methodology of social event such utilitarian data is called "target approval" in pharmaceutical industry speech. Created targets likewise incorporate those that the pharmaceutical business has had experience mounting medication revelation fights against before; such a history gives data on the synthetic practicality of building up a little sub-atomic restorative against the target and can give authorizing open doors and opportunity to-work markers regarding little atom remedial applicants.

As a rule, "new targets" are each one of those focuses on that are not "settled targets" yet which have been or are the subject of medication disclosure fights. These ordinarily incorporate newfound proteins, or proteins whose capacity has now ended up clear as an aftereffect of fundamental experimental exploration.

The larger part of targets at present chose for medication revelation endeavors are proteins. Two classes prevail: G-protein-coupled receptors (or GPCRs) and protein kinases.

Screening and design

The procedure of discovering another medication against a picked focus for a specific sickness normally includes high-throughput screening (HTS), wherein huge libraries of chemicals are tried for their capacity to change the target. For instance, if the target is a novel GPCR, mixes will be screened for their capacity to hinder or fortify that receptor (see adversary and agonist): if the target is a protein kinase, the chemicals will be tried for their capacity to repress that kinase.

An alternate critical capacity of HTS is to indicate how specific the mixes are for the picked target. The perfect is to discover a particle which will meddle with just the picked target, however not other, related targets. To this end, other screening runs will be made to see whether the "hits" against the picked target will meddle with other related targets - this is the procedure of cross-screening. Cross-screening is critical, on the grounds that the more disconnected focuses on a compound hits, the more probable that off-target toxicity will happen with that compound once it achieves the center.

It is improbable that a flawless medication competitor will rise up out of these early screening runs. It is all the more regularly watched that few mixes are found to have some level of action, and if these mixes offer basic synthetic gimmicks, one or more pharmacophores can then be produced. As of right now, restorative physicists will endeavor to utilize structure-action connections (SAR) to enhance certain peculiarities of the lead compound:

- increase activity against the chosen target
- reduce activity against unrelated targets

- improve the druglikeness or ADME properties of the molecule.

This methodology will require a few iterative screening runs, amid which, it is trusted, the properties of the new atomic elements will enhance, and permit the favored mixes to go ahead to in vitro and in vivo testing for action in the malady model of decision.

Amongst the physico-synthetic properties connected with medication ingestion incorporate ionization (pKa), and solvency; porousness can be dictated by PAMPA and Caco-2. PAMPA is appealing as an early screen because of the low utilization of medication and the minimal effort contrasted with tests, for example, Caco-2, gastrointestinal tract (GIT) and Blood–brain barrier (BBB) with which there is a high relationship.

A scope of parameters can be utilized to survey the nature of a compound, or a progression of mixes, as proposed in the Lipinski's Rule of Five. Such parameters incorporate computed properties, for example, cLogP to gauge lipophilicity, atomic weight, polar surface territory and measured properties, for example, intensity, in-vitro estimation of enzymatic leeway and so forth. A few descriptors, for example, ligand efficiency [13] (LE) and lipophilic efficiency[14][15] (LiPE) consolidate such parameters to survey drug likeness

While HTS is an ordinarily utilized technique for novel medication revelation, it is by all account not the only strategy. It is regularly conceivable to begin from a particle, which as of now has a portion of the sought properties. Such an atom may be extricated from a characteristic item or even be a medication available which could be enhanced (supposed "me as well" medications). Different techniques, for example, virtual high throughput screening, where screening is carried out utilizing PC produced models and endeavoring to "dock" virtual libraries to a target, are additionally regularly utilized

An alternate critical system for medication disclosure is medication plan, whereby the organic and physical properties of the target are concentrated on, and an expectation is made of the sorts of chemicals that may (e.g.) fit into a dynamic site. One case is part based lead revelation (FBLD). Novel pharmacophores can develop quickly from these activities. All in all, PC helped medication outline is regularly however not generally used to attempt to enhance the power and properties of new medication leads. When a lead compound arrangement has been created with sufficient target strength and selectivity and good medication like properties, maybe a couple mixes will then be proposed for medication advancement. The best of these is for the most part called the lead compound, while the other will be assigned as the "reinforcement".

Nature as source of drugs

Customarily numerous medications and different chemicals with natural action have been found by examining allelopathy - chemicals that creatures make that influence the movement of different life forms in the battle for survival. [16]

In spite of the ascent of combinatorial science as a fundamental piece of lead revelation process, regular items still assume a noteworthy part as beginning material for medication discovery.[17] A 2007 report[18] found that of the 974 little particle new synthetic elements grew somewhere around 1981 and 2006, 63% were characteristic inferred or semisynthetic subordinates of common items. For certain treatment regions, for example, antimicrobials, antineoplastics, antihypertensive and calming medications, the numbers were higher. Much of the time, these items have been utilized generally for a long time.

Regular items may be helpful as a wellspring of novel synthetic structures for present day strategies of improvement of antibacterial therapies.[19].Notwithstanding the inferred potential, just a small amount of Earth's living species has been tried for bioactivity.

Chemical diversity of natural products

As aforementioned, combinatorial science was a key innovation empowering the productive era of huge screening libraries for the needs of high-throughput screening. Then again, now, following two many years of combinatorial science, it has been brought up that notwithstanding the expanded proficiency in compound amalgamation, no increment in lead or medication applicants has been reached.[18] This has prompted examination of synthetic attributes of combinatorial science items, contrasted with existing medications or regular items. The chemoinformatics idea substance assorted qualities, portrayed as conveyance of mixes in the compound space in light of their physicochemical attributes, is regularly used to portray the distinction between the combinatorial science libraries and characteristic items. The manufactured, combinatorial library mixes appear to cover just a restricted and very uniform concoction space, while existing medications and especially regular items, display much more prominent substance differing qualities, disseminating all the more equally to the compound space.[17] The most unmistakable contrasts between characteristic items and mixes in combinatorial science libraries is the quantity of chiral focuses (much higher in common mixes), structure unbending nature (higher in regular mixes) and number of sweet-smelling moieties (higher in combinatorial science libraries). Other concoction contrasts between these two gatherings incorporate the way of heteroatoms (O and N improved in regular items, and S and halogen particles all the more regularly present in manufactured mixes), and level of non-sweet-smelling unsaturation (higher in characteristic items). As both structure inflexibility and chirality are both entrenched calculates therapeutic science known to improve mixes specificity and adequacy as a medication, it has been proposed that common items contrast great with today's combinatorial science libraries as potential lead atoms.

Natural product drug discovery

Two fundamental methodologies exist for the finding of new bioactive compound substances from characteristic sources.

The main is infrequently alluded to as irregular gathering and screening of material, yet indeed the accumulation is frequently a long way from arbitrary in that organic (regularly natural) information is utilized about which families show guarantee, in view of various variables, including past screening. This methodology is in light of the way that just a little part of earth's biodiversity has ever been tried for pharmaceutical action. It is additionally in view of the way that life forms living in an animal groups rich environment need to advance guarding and aggressive components to survive, systems which may conveniently be misused in the advancement of medications that can cure sicknesses influencing people. A gathering of plant, creature and microbial specimens from rich environments can possibly offer ascent to novel organic exercises worth misusing in the medication advancement process. One sample of a fruitful utilization of this methodology is the screening for antitumour operators by the National Cancer Institute, began in the 1960s. Paclitaxelwas recognized from Pacific yew tree Taxus brevifolia. Paclitaxel indicated against tumor movement by an already undescribed instrument (adjustment of microtubules) and is currently affirmed for clinical utilization for the treatment of lung, breast and ovarian malignancy, and additionally for Kaposi's sarcoma. Ahead of schedule in the 21st century, Cabazitaxel (made by Sanofi, a French firm), an alternate relative of taxol has been demonstrated viable against prostate tumor, additionally in light of the fact that it lives up to expectations by keeping the arrangement of microtubules, which pull the chromosomes separated in partitioning cells (such as cancer cells). Still another examples are:

1. Camptotheca (Camptothecin · Topotecan · Irinotecan · Rubitecan · Belotecan);
2. Podophyllum (Etoposide · Teniposide);
3. Anthracyclines (Aclarubicin · Daunorubicin · Doxorubicin · Epirubicin · Idarubicin · Amrubicin · Pirarubicin · Valrubicin · Zorubicin); 3b. Anthracenediones (Mitoxantrone · Pixantrone).

Nor do all drugs developed in this manner come from plants. Professor Louise Rollins-Smith of Vanderbilt University's Medical Center, for example, has developed from the skin of frogs a compound which blocks AIDS. Professor Rollins-Smith is aware of declining amphibian populations and has said: "We need to protect these species long enough for us to understand their medicinal cabinet." The second main approach involves Ethnobotany, the study of the general use of plants in society, and ethnopharmacology, an area inside ethnobotany, which is focused specifically on medicinal uses. Both of these two main approaches can be used in selecting starting materials for future drugs. Artemisinin, an antimalarial agent from sweet worm tree Artemisia annua, used in Chinese medicine since 200BC is one drug used as part of combination therapy for multiresistant Plasmodium falciparum.

Structural elucidation

The explanation of the concoction structure is discriminating to maintain a strategic distance from the re-disclosure of synthetic operators that is as of now known for its structure and substance movement. Mass spectrometry is a system in which individual mixes are recognized in view of their mass/charge degree, after ionization. Compound mixes exist in nature as mixtures, so the mix of fluid chromatography and mass spectrometry (LC-MS) is regularly used to particular the individual chemicals. Databases of mass spectras for known mixes are accessible, and can be utilized to allot a structure to an obscure mass range. Atomic attractive reverberation spectroscopy is the essential procedure for deciding synthetic structures of characteristic items. NMR yields data about individual hydrogen and carbon molecules in the structure, permitting definite reproduction of the atom's structural planning.

High Throughput Screening (HTS)

Introduction

High Throughput Screening (HTS) is a drug-discovery process widely used in the pharmaceutical industry. It leverages automation to quickly assay the biological or biochemical activity of a large number of drug-like compounds. It is a useful for discovering ligands for receptors, enzymes, ion-channels or other pharmacological targets, or pharmacologically profiling a cellular or biochemical pathway of interest. Typically, HTS assays are performed in "automation-friendly" microtiter plates with a 96, 384 or 1536 well format.

High throughput screen: an optimised, miniaturised assay format that enables the testing of > 100,000 chemically diverse compounds per day.

Assay: a test system in which biological activity can be detected

Hit: a molecule with confirmed concentration-dependent activity in a screen, and known chemical structure. The output of most screens

Progressible hit: a representative of a compound series with activity via acceptable mechanism of action and some limited structure-activity relationship information

Lead: a compound with potential (as measured by potency, selectivity, physico-chemical properties, absence of toxicity or novelty) to progress to a full drug development programme

Pharmacophore: minimal structure with essential features for activity
The life history of a successful drug

Drug discovery

Initial characterisation

Pre-clinical trials

Regulatory approval sought to start
trials in humans

Clinical trials Phases I, II, III

Submission of marketing/manufacturing
authorisation application to regulatory authorities

Regulatory authorities review
information and grant (or refuse) licences

Product goes on sale

Post-marketing surveillance

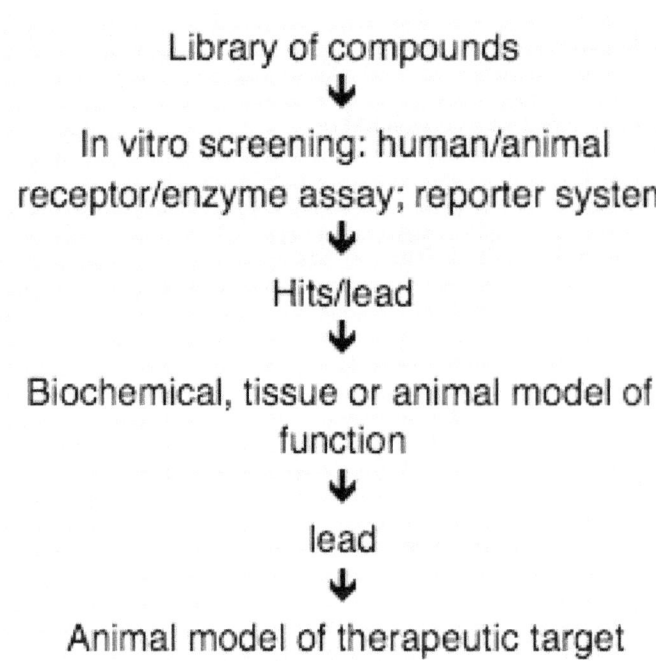

Library of compounds
↓
In vitro screening: human/animal
receptor/enzyme assay; reporter system
↓
Hits/lead
↓
Biochemical, tissue or animal model of
function
↓
lead
↓
Animal model of therapeutic target
↓
ADME, formulation, acute toxicology

High throughput screening for drug discovery

FACT 1: recent understanding of disease mechanisms has dramatically increased no. of protein targets for new drug treatment

FACT 2: new technologies have increased the no. of drugs that can be tested for activity at these targets.

high throughput screening (HTS) is 1° tool for early-stage drug discovery
HTS is process by which large nos. of compounds are rapidly tested for their ability to modify the properties of a selected biological target.
Goal is to identify 'hits' or 'leads'
 - affect target in desired manner
 - active at fairly low concs (\ more likely to show specificity)
 - new structure
The greater the no. and diversity of compounds screened, the more successful screen is likely to be.
HTS = 50,000-100,000 cpds screened per day!!!

Goals and limitations of HTS

Aim of screening is to find progressible hits, not to discover the lead molecule itself

The majority of drug targets are

a) G-protein coupled 7 TM receptors (est total 5000)

b) nuclear receptors (est total >150)

c) ion channels (est total 1000)

d) enzymes (est total uncertain)

Take top 100 drugs   - 18 bind to GPCR

- 10 bind to nuclear receptors

- 16 bind to ion channels

- most of remainder inhibit enzymes

Knowledge gained from one drug target can be transferred to related targets. e.g molecular technology required to work with 1 GPCR is useful for other GPCRs, including cloning and expression systems and info on structure and ligands.

HTS can be used to screen for activity at all of these targets.

Activity =   (a) potency

(b) specificity, if screen simultaneously against different targets

Implementation of HTS

Need 4 elements:

Assay plate preparation

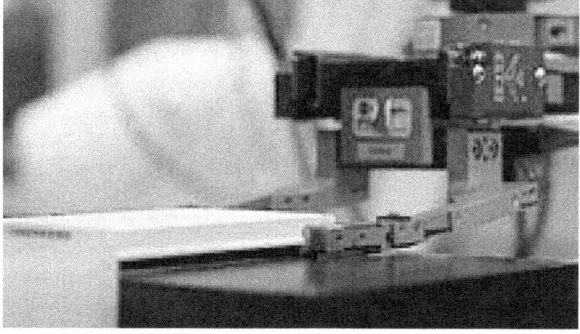

A robot arm handles an assay plate

The key labware or testing vessel of HTS is the microtiter plate: a little holder, normally dispensable and made of plastic, that peculiarities a lattice of little, open divots called wells. By and large, cutting edge (around 2013) microplates for HTS have either 384, 1536, or 3456 wells. These are all products of 96, mirroring the first 96-well microplate with divided wells of 8 x 12 9 mm . The majority of the wells contain tentatively valuable matter, contingent upon the way of the investigation. This could be a watery arrangement of dimethyl sulfoxide (DMSO) and some other synthetic intensify, the last of which varies for every well over the plate. It could likewise contain cells or proteins of some sort. (Alternate wells may be vacant or contain untreated examples, proposed for utilization as exploratory controls.)

A screening office regularly holds a library of stock plates, whose substance are painstakingly recorded, and each of which may have been made by the lab or acquired from a business source. These stock plates themselves are not straightforwardly utilized as a part of investigations; rather, separate test plates are made as required. An examine plate is basically a duplicate of a stock plate, made by pipetting a little measure of fluid (frequently measured in nanoliters) from the wells of a stock plate to the relating wells of a totally void plate.

1) suitable libraries of compounds

Source of chemicals for screen:
- in-house collection (5×10^5 - 10^6) of diverse samples.
- supplement by acquisitions from specialist companies
- combinatorial chemistry allows synthesis of large no of diverse molecules.

Reaction observation

To plan for a measure, the analyst fills every well of the plate with some legitimate element that he wishes to lead the investigation upon, for example, a protein, cells, or a creature incipient organism. After some brooding time has gone to permit the natural matter to ingest, tie to, or generally respond (or neglect to respond) with the mixes in the wells, estimations are taken over all the plate's wells, either physically or by a machine. Manual estimations are regularly vital when the scientist is utilizing microscopy to (for instance) look for changes or deserts in embryonic advancement created by the wells' mixes, searching for impacts that a PC couldn't without much of a stretch focus independent from anyone else. Something else, a specific mechanized examination machine can run various analyses on the wells, (for example, sparkling captivated light on them and measuring reflectivity, which can be a sign of protein tying). For this situation, the machine yields the consequence of every test as a lattice of numeric qualities, with every number mapping to the worth acquired from a solitary well. A high-limit investigation machine can quantify many plates in the space of a couple of minutes like this, creating a huge number of test data points rapidly.

Contingent upon the aftereffects of this first test, the analyst can perform catch up examines inside the same screen by "carefully choosing" fluid from the source wells that gave intriguing results (known as "hits") into new examine plates, and afterward re-running the trial to gather further information on this contracted set, affirming and refining perceptions.

Automation systems

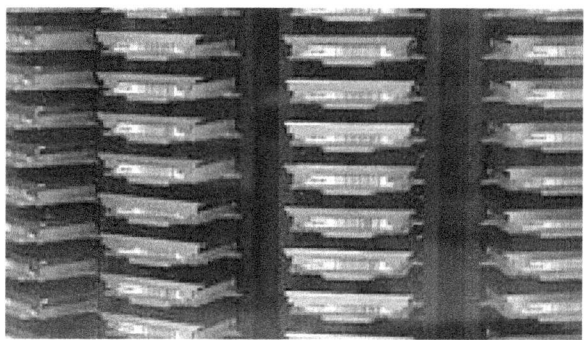

A carousel system to store assay plates for high storage capacity and high speed access

Computerization is an imperative component in HTS's helpfulness. Commonly, an incorporated robot framework comprising of one or more robots transports examine microplates from station to station for test and reagent expansion, blending, brooding, lastly readout or location. A HTS framework can typically get ready, brood, and investigate numerous plates at the same time, further speeding the information accumulation process. HTS robots that can test up to 100,000 mixes every day right now exist.[20] Automatic settlement pickers pick a large number of microbial states for high throughput hereditary screening.[21] The term uHTS or ultra-high-throughput screening alludes (around 2008) to screening in overabundance of 100,000 mixes every day.

2) assay method configured for automation

Assay requirements:

a) pharmacology of the target should not be altered by the molecular manipulations

b) cost of assay development and reagents low

c) easy to use and suitable for automation and miniaturisation. Use multi-well plates: 96, 192, 384, 864, 1536 and assay requiring few manipulations, no plate-o-plate transfers or washing steps

d) robust signal-to-noise ratio. Hit defined as activity above a certain threshold

 e.g. K_i < 5 nM

   Emax >30% increase over basal

e) ideally be non-radioactive

Often express target genes in appropriate host systems

 e.g. bacterial, yeast, viral, invertebrate and mammalian cells.

a) Radioligand binding assays

• Measures affinity of library compounds for target.

• Need high affinity radioligand that binds to site of interest and cells transfected with target site.

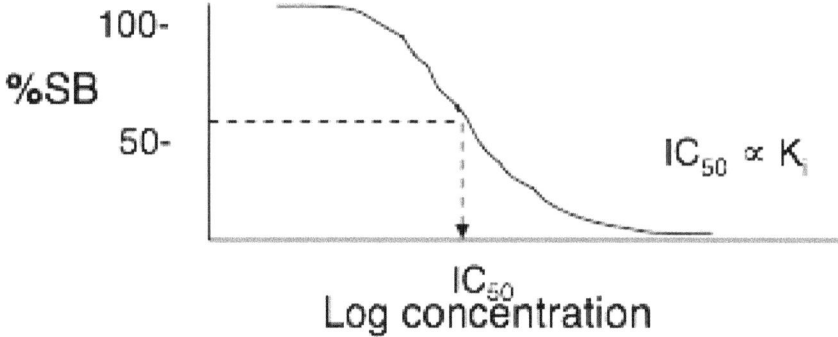

• measure competitive displacement of radioligand from target site

• Specificity can be assessed by including other possible targets in screen

èrelative affinity for multiple sites

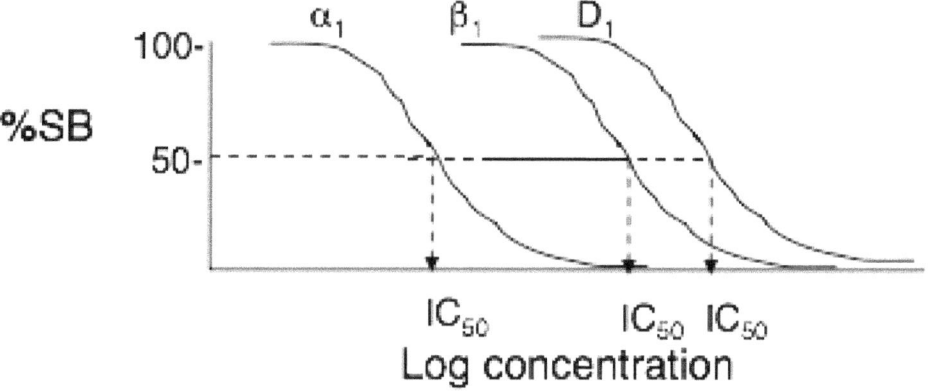

PROBLEM: hard to miniaturise radioactive assays (counting takes too long). Alternative is to use fluorescence techniques.

(b) Cell-based fluorescence and radiotracer assays

Useful for measuring ion-channel function

e.g.measure movement of Ca^{2+} in a fluorescent-imaging plate-reader (FLIPR)

 • cells are loaded with the fluorescent Ca^{2+} indicator Fluo-3

 • depolarisation with high KCl activates Ca^{2+} channels and allows Ca^{2+} entry

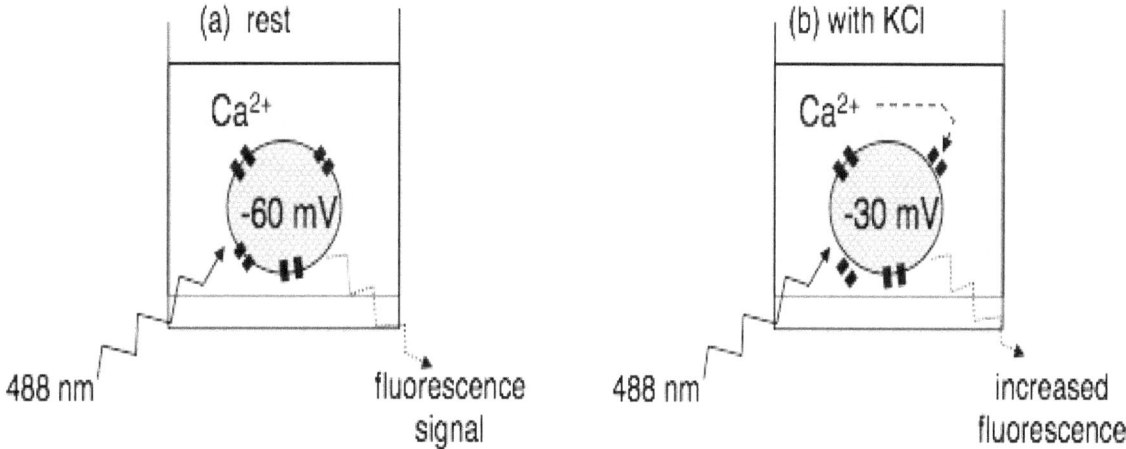

c) melanophore assays

Melanophores = pigmented cells derived from neural crest. Prepare immortalised melanophores from *Xenopus laevis*

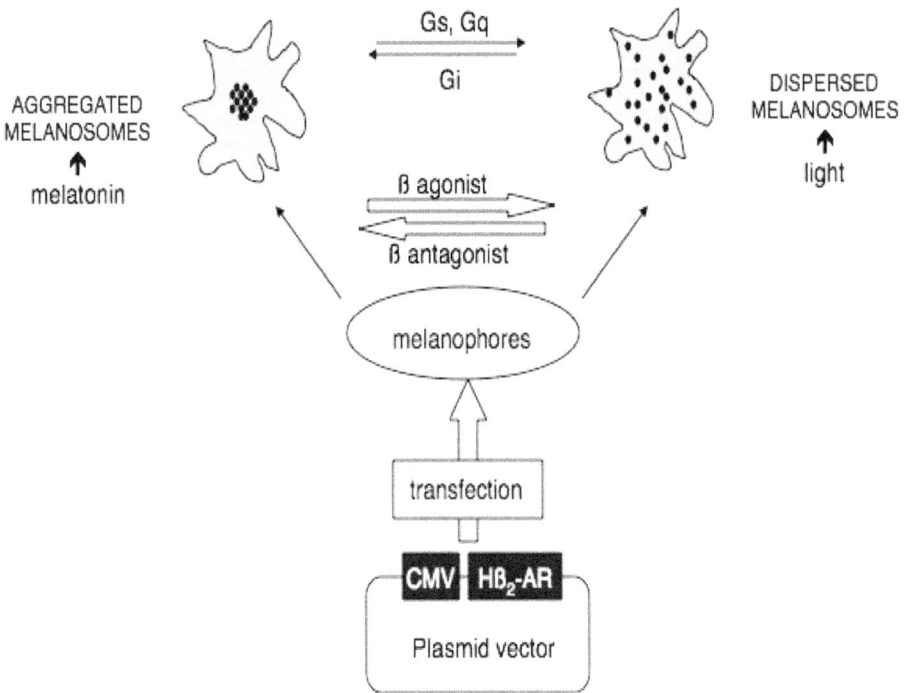

(d) Reporter gene assays

Rather than measure the immediate cellular response, it may be easier to measure the subsequent transcriptional change

isoprenaline binding to ß-adrenceptors

ê

á cAMP

ê

PKA activation and translocation to nucleus

ê

phosphorylation of transcription factor CREB that recognises cAMP response elements

(CREs)

ê

á expression of reporter gene whose transcription is driven by an enhancer containing CREs

ê

Measure reporter gene product in HTS format

• Examples of reporter genes: ß-galactosidase; luciferase; alkaline phosphatase; green fluorescent protein.

• Useful for measuring responses from Gi, Gs or Gq-coupled receptors

e) Cell viability assays

f) Cell proliferation assays

All screens have danger of false negatives and false positives

     Not such a problem   waste time and resources

HTS is less useful for evaluating - bioavailability - - pharmackinetics

 - toxicity

 - absolute specificity

3) Robotics workstation

• Robots handle assays in multi-well formats.

 - sample dilutions

 - sample dispensing

 - plate washing (more problematic with higher well density (844- and 1536-well plates))

Hard to automate cell lysis or permeabilisation steps (necessary for many 2nd messenger responses).

• Full automation allows 24 h continuous operation without requiring shift work.

• More efficient and economical.

Experimental design and data analysis

With the capacity of quick screening of various mixes, (for example, little particles or siRNAs) to recognize dynamic mixes, HTS has prompted a blast in the rate of information created lately .[22]Consequently, a standout amongst the most principal difficulties in HTS examinations is to gather biochemical hugeness from hills of information, which depends on the improvement and reception of suitable trial outlines and investigative systems for both quality control and hit choice .[23] HTS exploration is one of the fields that have a peculiarity portrayed by John Blume, Chief Science Officer for Applied Proteomics, Inc., as takes after: Soon, if a researcher does not see a few measurements or simple information taking care of advancements, he or she may not be thought to be a genuine sub-atomic scientist and, therefore, will basically turn into "a dinosaur."[24]

4) computerized data handling system

A great deal of data is generated. Must be accurate and reproducible.

 Need good computerised data handling systems.

Which strategy is best for hit identification?

When a target is identified, a decision has to be made about which chemicals to screen, in order to identify potential lead compounds.

Random screening

All possible drug molecules screened against target.

Estimated no. of possible drug molecules is $\pm 10^{40}$!!!

This is simply not possible.

Focused screening

A limited number of compounds are pre-selected for screening.

Has proved successful as a hit generation strategy.

Useful when 3D structure of target is known (e.g. crystal structure of a receptor)

- use computer modeling to predict optimal structure to interact with target

- use known ligand to construct 3D pharmacophore

In either case, select compounds from library or design new compounds and screen.

Focused screening will find novel hits BUT the required information may not be available.

Diversity screening

The aim is to synthesize, access and test all the molecules that could be drug candidates.

How many diverse samples should be tested???

Glaxo suggest a sample set of up to 500,000 molecules è HTS

Diversity screening will find unexpected hits and generate data for SAR.

Focused and diversity screens can be run in parallel.

Virtual Screening

The medications grew in the previous 100 years are found to connect with give or take 500 focuses; in the same period, about 20,000,000 natural mixes including common items have been orchestrated or confined. Besides, the genomic and useful genomic undertakings have created extra 1500 druggable focuses for medication mediation to control human sicknesses (21). Consequently, it is trustworthy that an expansive number of new drugs, in any event numerous leads or hits, stow away in the current synthetic mine. Be that as it may, how to scrape out this source is a hard errand. Gathering all the current mixes and screening them haphazardly against all the potential focuses on one by one are greatly strange, in light of the fact that it is painfully lavish and time intensive. Be that as it may, virtual screening demonstrates a dawning to fulfill this necessity. In reality, virtual screening has been included into the pipeline of medication revelation as a functional instrument (22). Basically, virtual screening is intended for looking largescale speculative databases of compound structures or virtual libraries by utilizing computational examination for selecting a constrained number of applicant particles prone to be dynamic against a picked organic receptor (23). Along these lines, virtual screening is a consistent augmentation of 3-D pharmacophore-based database seeking (PBDS) (24) or atomic docking (25), which is skilled of naturally assessing vast databases of mixes. Two techniques have been utilized as a part of virtual screening (see Fig. 3): 1) utilizing PBDS to recognize potential hits from the databases, for the most part in the cases that 3-D structures of the targets are obscure also, 2) utilizing sub-atomic docking way to rank the databases if the 3-D structures of the targets are accessible. Ordinarily, these two methodologies are utilized simultaneously or consecutively, since the previous can channel out the mixes rapidly and the recent can assess the ligand-receptor tying all the more precisely. For the pharmacophore-based screening, a 3-D-pharmacophore highlight is developed by structure-action relationship investigation on a progression of dynamic exacerbates (26) or is reasoned from the X-beam precious stone structure of a ligand-receptor complex (27). Taking this 3-D–pharmacophore emphasize as an inquiry structure, 3-D database pursuit can be performed to choose the atoms from the accessible compound databases, which contain the pharmacophore components and may comply with the pharmacophore geometric limitations. At that point the chose mixes are acquired either from business sources or from natural amalgamation for the genuine pharmacologic measures (see Fig. 3). Docking-based virtual screening (DBVS) requires the structural data of both receptors and mixes. The general strategy of DBVS incorporates five stages: receptor displaying (virtual screening mode development), compound database era, PC screening, hit atoms post processing, what's more, test bioassay. The center venture of virtual screening is docking and scoring. Docking is a methodology to place every particle from a 3-D little atom database into the tying site of a receptor protein, streamline the relative introduction furthermore, conformity for a ligand collaborating with a protein, furthermore, select atoms from the database that may tie to the protein hard. Billions of conceivable conformities can be made for an adaptable ligand even with a couple of flexibility degrees in the revolution space alone, current advancement calculations can't test comprehensively for all conformities and introductions, evidently to record for the adaptability of protein with a great many degrees of opportunity. Accordingly, as opposed to seeking comprehensively in the pursuit space, an advancement calculation should test the arrangements viably and quickly near to the worldwide ideal (28). Fundamentally, the advancement calculations utilized generally by atomic docking system can be isolated into three classifications: numerical advancement routines, irregular then again stochastic routines, and half and half streamlining strategies. Basically, there are three sorts of scoring capacities (29), which incorporate power field based scoring capacities, exact scoring capacities, and information based scoring capacities. Nonetheless, no single scoring capacity can perform acceptably for each framework on the grounds that numerous physical phenomena deciding sub-atomic distinguishment were not completely represented, for example, entropic alternately dissolvable impacts (13). Since Kuntz et al. (30) distributed the first and foremost docking calculation DOCK in 1982, more than 20 docking projects have been created in late two decades. Of the current docking system, DOCK, FlexX, AutoDock, and GOLD are most oftentimes utilized, different projects, for example, Glide, ICM, what's more, Surflex have been connected effectively in virtual screening. In any case, numerous constraints difficulties still exist for atomic docking, for example, exact expectation of the coupling conformity and liking, protein adaptability, entropy, and dissolvable impacts. Without uncertainty, the atomic docking methodology is still an intricate and testing task of computational science what's more, science (25, 31). Virtual screening has found various dynamic mixes what's more, leads, more than 50 mixes have gone into clinical trials, and some have been endorsed as medications (2). Virtual screening advanced the hit rate (characterized as the remainder in rate of the quantity of dynamic mixes at a specific focus partitioned by the quantity of all mixes tentatively tried) by around 100-fold to 1000-fold over arbitrary screening (22, 32). Also, virtual screening gives an option route in fleetly discovering new leads of a few targets, though the systems for high-throughput screening stay being developed (e.g. potassium particle (K+) channels). By utilizing docking-based virtual screening in conjunction with electrophysiological test, we found 10 new blockers of the eukaryotic Shaker K+ channels, 4 characteristic item blockers (33), and 6 manufactured exacerbates (34).

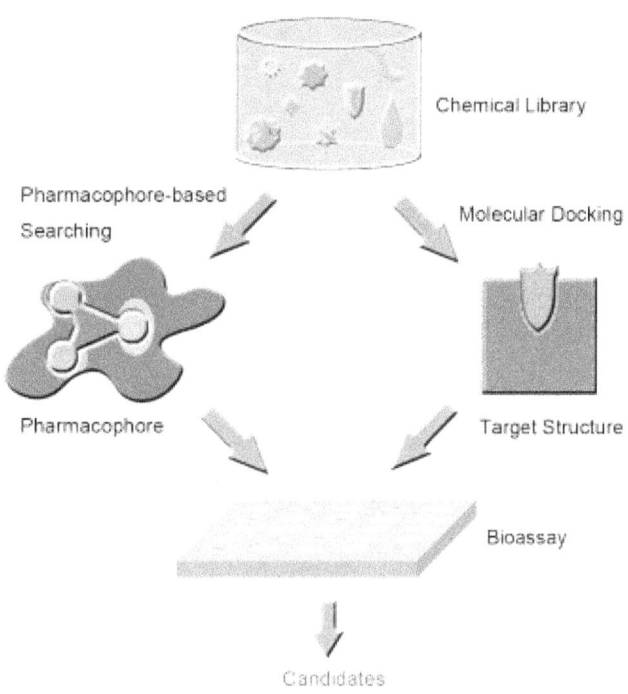

Figure 3   The flowchart for virtual screening.

Quality control

Great HTS measures are discriminating in HTS tests. The improvement of amazing HTS tests requires the mix of both test and computational methodologies for quality control (QC). Three imperative method for QC are (i) great plate plan, (ii) the determination of successful positive and negative substance/natural controls, and (iii) the improvement of viable QC measurements to gauge the level of separation so that measures with second rate information quality can be recognized. [25] A decent plate configuration serves to distinguish deliberate mistakes (particularly those connected with well position) and figure out what standardization ought to be utilized to evacuate/decrease the effect of methodical blunders on both QC and hit selection.[23]

Compelling diagnostic QC routines serve as a guardian for magnificent quality tests. In a run of the mill HTS test, an agreeable refinement between a positive control and a negative reference, for example, a negative control is a file for good quality. Numerous quality-appraisal measures have been proposed to gauge the level of separation between a positive control and a negative reference. Sign to-foundation degree, sign to-clamor proportion, signal window, examine variability proportion, and Z-variable have been received to assess information quality. [23] [26] Strictly institutionalized mean contrast (SSMD) has as of late been proposed for evaluating information quality in HTS tests. [27] [28]

HIT To Lead

Hit selection

Hit to lead (H2L) otherwise called lead era is a stage in right on time drug revelation where little atom hits from a high throughput screen (HTS) are assessed and experience restricted advancement to distinguish guaranteeing lead compounds.[37] These lead mixes experience more broad improvement in a consequent venture of medication disclosure called lead Optimixation (LO).[38][39] The medication disclosure handle by and large takes after the accompanying way that incorporates a hit to lead stage:

- target validation (TV) → assay development → high-throughput screening → hit to lead (H2L) → lead optimization (LO) → preclinical drug development → clinical drug development

The hit to lead stage begins with affirmation and assessment of the introductory screening hits and is trailed by amalgamation of analogs (hit development). Normally the starting screening hits presentation tying affinities for their organic focus in the micromolar ($10{-}6$ molar fixation) range. Through constrained H2L advancement, the affinities of the hits are frequently enhanced by a few requests of greatness to the nanomolar ($10{-}9$ M) range. The hits additionally experience restricted improvement to enhance metabolic half life so that the mixes can be tried in creature models of malady furthermore to enhance selectivity against other organic targets tying that may bring about undesirable sympt

Hit confirmation

After hits are identified from a high throughput screen, the hits are confirmed and evaluated using the following methods:

• Re-testing: compounds that were discovered dynamic against the chose target are re-tried utilizing the same examine conditions utilized amid the HTS.

• Dose reaction bend era: a few compound focuses are tried utilizing the same examine, an IC50 or EC50 worth is then created.

• Orthogonal testing: Confirmed hits are examined utilizing an alternate measure which is normally closer to the target physiological condition or utilizing an alternate innovation.

• Secondary screening: Confirmed hits are tried in a useful measure or in a cell situation. Film penetrability is typically a basic parameter.

• Chemical managability: Medicinal scientific experts assess mixes as per their union possibility and different parameters, for example, up-scaling or expenses

• Biophysical testing: Nuclear attractive reverberation (NMR), Isothermal Titration Calorimetry, element light disseminating, surface plasmon reverberation, double polarization interferometry, microscale thermophoresis (MST) are normally used to survey whether the compound ties viably to the focus on, the stoïchiometry of tying, any related conformational change and to recognize unbridled inhibitors.

• Hit positioning and bunching: Confirmed hit mixes are then positioned as per the different hit affirmation tests.

• Freedom to work assessment: Hit compound structures are immediately weighed in particular databases to figure out whether they are patentable[40]

Hit expansion

Following hit confirmation, several compound clusters will be chosen according to their characteristics in the previously defined tests. An Ideal compound cluster will:

- have compound members that exhibit a high affinity towards the target (less than 1 μM)
- Moderate molecular weight and lipophilicity (usually measured as cLogP). Affinity, molecular weight and lipophilicity can be linked in single parameter such as ligand efficiency and lipophilic efficiency to assess druglikeness
- show chemical tractability
- be free of Intellectual property
- not interfere with the P450 enzymes nor with the P-glycoproteins
- not bind to human serum albumin
- be soluble in water (above 100 μM)
- be stable
- have a good druglikeness
- exhibit cell membrane permeability
- show significant biological activity in a cellular assay
- not exhibit cytotoxicity

- not be metabolized rapidly
- show selectivity versus other related targets

The venture group will normally choose somewhere around three and six compound arrangement to be further investigated. The following step will permit the testing of similar to mixes to characterize Quantitative structure-movement relationship (QSAR). Analogs can be immediately chosen from an interior library or obtained from financially accessible sources. Restorative physicists will likewise begin combining related mixes utilizing diverse routines, for example, combinatorial science, high-throughput science or more classical organic science blend.

A compound with a coveted size of impacts in a HTS screen is known as a hit. The procedure of selecting hits is called hit choice. The systematic techniques for hit choice in screens without reproduces (normally in essential screens) contrast from those with recreates (generally in affirming screens). Case in point, the z-score technique is suitable for screens without recreates though the t-measurement is suitable for screens with repeats. The estimation of SSMD for screens without imitates likewise varies from that for screens with duplicates.[23]

For hit determination in essential screens without imitates, the effectively interpretable ones are normal fold change, mean distinction, percent restraint, and percent action. On the other hand, they don't catch information variability successfully. The z-score technique orSSMD, which can catch information variability taking into account a presumption that each compound has the same variability as a negative reference in the screens [29] .[30] However, exceptions are basic in HTS analyses, and techniques, for example, z-score are delicate to anomalies and can be risky. As a result, hearty techniques, for example, the z*-score technique, SSMD*, B-score strategy, and quantile-based system have been proposed and received for hit determination. [23] [31] [32]

In a screen with reproduces, we can specifically gauge variability for every compound; as a result, we ought to utilize SSMD or t-measurement that does not depend on the solid supposition that the z-score and z*-score depend on. One issue with the utilization of t-measurement and related p-qualities is that they are influenced by both specimen size and impact size.[33] They originate from testing for no mean contrast, and along these lines are not intended to quantify the span of compound impacts. For hit choice, the real investment is the span of impact in a tried compound. SSMD straightforwardly surveys the extent of effects.[34] SSMD has additionally been demonstrated to be superior to other regularly utilized impact sizes .[35] The populace estimation of SSMD is practically identical crosswise over examinations and, therefore, we can utilize the same cutoff for the populace estimation of SSMD to gauge the measure of compound impacts .[36]

Techniques for increased throughput and efficiency

Interesting circulations of mixes over one or numerous plates can be utilized either to expand the quantity of tests every plate or to decrease the difference of measure results, or both. The improving presumption made in this methodology is that any N mixes in the same well won't regularly interface with one another, or the measure focus, in a way that generally changes the capacity of the test to identify genuine hits.

Case in point, envision a plate wherein aggravate An is in wells 1-2-3, compound B is in wells 2-3-4, and compound C is in wells 3-4-5. In a measure of this plate against a given focus on, a hit in wells 2, 3, and 4 would show that compound B is the in all likelihood specialists, while likewise giving three estimations of exacerbate B's viability against the predetermined target. Business utilizations of this methodology include blends in which no two mixes ever impart more than one well, to diminish the (second-arrange) probability of obstruction between sets of mixes being screened.

Recent advances

In March 2010, examination was distributed showing a HTS methodology permitting 1,000 times speedier screening (100 million responses in 10 hours) at 1-millionth the expense (utilizing 10−7 times the reagent volume) than routine procedures utilizing drop-based microfluidics.[18] Drops of liquid divided by oil supplant microplate wells and permit investigation and hit sorting while reagents are coursing through channels.

In 2010, scientists added to a silicon sheet of lenses that can be put over microfluidic exhibits to permit the fluorescence estimation of 64 diverse yield channels all the while with a solitary camera.[19] This procedure can investigate 200,000 drops every second.

Lead Optimization phase

The target of this medication revelation stage is to blend lead mixes, new analogs with enhanced intensity, diminished off-target exercises, and physiochemical/metabolic properties suggestive of sensible in vivo pharmacokinetics. This enhancement is proficient through concoction adjustment of the hit structure, with alterations picked by utilizing learning of the structure-action relationship (SAR) and in addition structure-based outline if structural data about the target is accessible.

Candidate Drug

A compound (small molecules, neutralizer, and so forth.) with solid restorative potential and whose movement and specificity have been advanced. The purpose of flight for crucial analysts (essential and scholastic examination) comprises in recognizing and approving restorative targets prone to be included in a given infection. When the target has been recognized, portrayed and approved by a progression of natural tests, it is important to recognize the substances equipped for following up on the target (actuation, hindrance) properly. Dynamic atoms are recognized by screening and are called "hits". At that point new tests are performed to quantify their dosage impact and physicochemical properties. PC displaying of the compound structure of the hits and their communication with the target licenses outlining new subsidiaries that experience new tests to gauge the restorative capability of these particles and their ability to be managed to people. Therapeutic science subsequently improves the action of these particles on the target and their conduct in vivo (harmfulness, bioavailability, and so on.). Accordingly lead particles are acquired. After a few cycles of streamlining (trades between displaying, concoction combination and natural tests), the substance introducing ideal attributes is picked as an applicant medication. This substance is then subjected to another arrangement of tests, and preclinical and clinical trials.

Developability evaluation has ended up regular practice over the pharmaceutical business to highlight key biopharmaceutical properties that recognize lead mixes from advancement competitors. Evaluating developability orders dangers and difficulties for opportune advancement and conveyance of new substance substances and permits the determination of the best medication competitor with an ideal harmony in the middle of pharmacological and medication like properties, while as yet paying consideration on conveying a safe improvement applicant. Numerous logical orders are included in surveying developability over the pharmaceutical business including therapeutic science, revelation science, pharmaceutical sciences, drug digestion system and pharmacokinetics (PK), and toxicology. Be that as it may, instead of only concentrating on developability evaluation in each of these controls and in segregation, the Drug Candidate Selection center gathering (DCSFG) will offer an incorporated and cross-disciplinary view on evaluating developability for compound choice and improvement, much in accordance with how it is really evaluated in the pharmaceutical business.

Goals

- Engage focus group membership via a survey to solicit ideas/input for DCSFG goals.
- Develop programming for future AAPS meetings in collaboration with other AAPS focus groups on topics aimed at producing successful clinical candidates that, in addition to being efficacious and safe, also have good physicochemical, absorption, distribution, metabolism, excretion, and PK properties.
- Compose an article showcasing the new focus group and a developability topic in the *AAPS Newsmagazine* or the DDDI section newsletter.
- Explore collaboration with other societies on developability programming—for example with the American Chemical Society on candidate selection criteria.

Drug Candidate Selection

One of the essential ventures in medication advancement is the determination of the most ideal clinical competitor, i.e. the NCE/NBE with the most obvious opportunity with regards to clinical achievement. For this reason in vitro and in vivo studies are led to allow further choice of lead medication applicants with alluring retention, appropriation, digestion system, discharge, toxicology (ADMET) properties and also pharmacology and adequacy to help in the expectation of clinical 'medication like' properties. Fulfillment of the medication competitor choice studies will give the information to backing the designation to 'clinical applicant' of the best compound inside a rundown of potential applicants. It is vital to kill potential medication competitors that are prone to fizzle in clinical trials as ahead of schedule as would be prudent in their advancement ('Fail quick and modest').

There is no standard medication competitor choice system and the achievement of such a project is established on the nature of the inquiries that are asked. What data is required for a particular compound, with particular concoction physical attributes and a particular clinical sign and/or clinical necessities?

Officially in such early stage a decent target item profile is obliged to have the capacity to direct the vital inquiries to be asked. Basically a stage savvy methodology is taken in the choice of the perfect clinical hopeful, with (particularly in the early ventures of determination) clear go-no go measure.

Drug Consultant has planned different hopeful determination programs for distinctive sorts of items. In light of that experience Drug Consultant can help you with asking the right inquiries, advancement of your project or give a second assessment (hole investigation) on the took after choice system and the choices taken. Have the information been assessed appropriately and have the right mixes been chosen for the following step?

With the introduction of high-throughput screening in the early 1990s into drug discovery and preclinical screening of candidate molecules, the pharmaceutical industry had high hopes of finding new molecules for specific targets at a faster rate. On a daily basis, thousands of compounds could be tested with regard to their affinity to target receptors and other possible binding sites, such as specific metabolizing enzymes or similar receptors located on other organs. This not only opened the door to select new and more specific compounds, but also helped to select and dispose of compounds with properties deemed undesirable. In fact, one may argue that the latter has become the main use of high-throughout screening, as more and more stringent criteria have been added to the hurdles that a new molecule must pass before being tested in preclinical settings and animal models. Thus, compounds that are found to be mainly metabolized by any major cytochrome P-450 enzymes or enzymes that show polymorphism, can induce enzymes, are substrates of the glycoprotein family of receptors, have low or moderate affinity to the target receptor and many other arbitrary, prespecified criteria, have a very low chance of making it past the screening stage. Such strict selection criteria prevent clinical, and hence costly, development of drugs that presumably have a high risk of failure further down the development road. However, it also excludes potentially good drug candidates from entering the preclinical phase of development.

The process of eliminating a drug candidate does not end with entry to animal testing. By contrast, any sign of undesired properties in animals could cause termination of investigation into the molecule. As an example, a short elimination half-life in rats or dogs is often considered an undesired property of the compound and could result in termination of its development. Another example would be low bioavailability in the tested animal models.

References:

1.Anson D, Ma J, He J-Q (1 May 2009). "Identifying Cardiotoxic Compounds". Genetic Engineering & Biotechnology News. TechNote **29** (9) (Mary Ann Liebert). pp. 34–35. ISSN 1935-472X. OCLC 77706455. Archived from the original on 25 July 2009. Retrieved 25 July 2009.

2.Paul SM, Mytelka DS, Dunwiddie CT, Persinger CC, Munos BH, Lindborg SR, Schacht AL (March 2010). "How to improve R&D productivity: the pharmaceutical industry's grand challenge". Nat Rev Drug Discov **9** (3): 203–14. doi:10.1038/nrd3078. PMID 20168317

3. Warren J (2011). "Drug discovery: lessons from evolution". Br J Clin Pharmacol **71** (4): 497–503. doi:10.1111/j.1365-2125.2010.03854.x. PMC 3080636. PMID 21395642.

4. Rask-Andersen M, Almén MS, Schiöth HB (August 2011). "Trends in the exploitation of novel drug targets.". Nature Reviews Drug Discovery **8** (10): 549–90. doi:10.1038/nrd3478. PMID 21804595

13. Hopkins AL, Groom CR, Alex A (May 2004). "Ligand efficiency: a useful metric for lead selection". Drug Discov. Today **9** (10): 430–1. doi:10.1016/S1359-6446(04)03069-7. PMID 15109945.

14. Ryckmans T, Edwards MP, Horne VA, Correia AM, Owen DR, Thompson LR, Tran I, Tutt MF, Young T (August 2009). "Rapid assessment of a novel series of selective CB(2) agonists using parallel synthesis protocols: A Lipophilic Efficiency (LipE) analysis". Bioorg. Med. Chem. Lett. **19** (15): 4406–9. doi:10.1016/j.bmcl.2009.05.062. PMID 19500981

15. Leeson PD, Springthorpe B (November 2007). "The influence of drug-like concepts on decision-making in medicinal chemistry". Nat Rev Drug Discov **6** (11): 881–90. doi:10.1038/nrd2445. PMID 17971784

16. Roger, Manuel Joaquín Reigosa; Reigosa, Manuel J.; Pedrol, Nuria; González, Luís (2006), Allelopathy: a physiological process with ecological implications, Springer, p. 1, ISBN 1-4020-4279-5

17. Feher M, Schmidt JM (2003). "Property distributions: differences between drugs, natural products, and molecules from combinatorial chemistry". J Chem Inf Comput Sci **43** (1): 218–27. doi:10.1021/ci0200467. PMID 12546556

18. Newman DJ, Cragg GM (March 2007). "Natural products as sources of new drugs over the last 25 years". J. Nat. Prod. **70** (3): 461–77. doi:10.1021/np068054v. PMID 17309302

19. von Nussbaum F, Brands M, Hinzen B, Weigand S, Häbich D (August 2006). "Antibacterial natural products in medicinal chemistry--exodus or revival?". Angew. Chem. Int. Ed. Engl. **45** (31): 5072–129. doi:10.1002/anie.200600350. PMID 16881035. "The handling of natural products is cumbersome, requiring nonstandardized workflows and extended timelines. Revisiting natural products with modern chemistry and target-finding tools from biology (reversed genomics) is one option for their revival."

20. Hann MM, Oprea TI (June 2004). "Pursuing the leadlikeness concept in pharmaceutical research". Curr Opin **8** (3): 255–63. doi:10.1016/j.cbpa.2004.04.003. PMID 15183323

21. http://peds.oxfordjournals.org/content/20/7/327.abstract

22. Howe D, Costanzo M, Fey P, Gojobori T, Hannick L, Hide W, Hill DP, Kania R, Schaeffer M, Pierre SS, Twigger S, White O, Rhee SY (2008). "Big data: The future of biocuration". Nature **455** (7209): 47–50. Bibcode:2008Natur.455...47H. doi:10.1038/455047a. PMC 2819144. PMID 18769432

23. Zhang XHD (2011). Optimal High-Throughput Screening: Practical Experimental Design and Data Analysis for Genome-scale RNAi Research. Cambridge University Press. ISBN 978-0-521-73444-8.

24. Eisenstein M (2006). "Quality control". Nature **442** (7106): 1067–70. Bibcode:2006Natur.442.1067E. doi:10.1038/4421067a. PMID 16943838

25. Zhang XHD, Espeseth AS, Johnson EN, Chin J, Gates A, Mitnaul LJ, Marine SD, Tian J, Stec EM, Kunapuli P, Holder DJ, Heyse JF, Strulocivi B, Ferrer M (2008). "Integrating experimental and analytic approaches to improve data quality in genome-scale RNAi screens". Journal of Biomolecular Screening **13** (5): 378–89. doi:10.1177/1087057108317145. PMID 18480473

26. Zhang JH, Chung TDY, Oldenburg KR (1999). "A simple statistical parameter for use in evaluation and validation of high throughput screening assays". Journal of Biomolecular Screening **4** (2): 67–73. doi:10.1177/108705719900400206. PMID 10838414

27. Zhang, XHD (2007). "A pair of new statistical parameters for quality control in RNA interference high-throughput screening assays". Genomics **89** (4): 552–61. doi:10.1016/j.ygeno.2006.12.014. PMID 17276655

28. Zhang XHD (2008). "Novel analytic criteria and effective plate designs for quality control in genome-scale RNAi screens". Journal of Biomolecular Screening **13** (5): 363–77. doi:10.1177/1087057108317062. PMID 18567841

29. Zhang XHD (2007). "A new method with flexible and balanced control of false negatives and false positives for hit selection in RNA interference high-throughput screening assays". Journal of Biomolecular Screening **12** (5): 645–55. doi:10.1177/1087057107300645. PMID 17517904

30. Zhang XHD, Ferrer M, Espeseth AS, Marine SD, Stec EM, Crackower MA, Holder DJ, Heyse JF, Strulovici B (2007). "The use of strictly standardized mean difference for hit selection in primary RNA interference high-throughput screening experiments". Journal of Biomolecular Screening **12** (4): 645–55. doi:10.1177/1087057107300646

31. Zhang XHD, Yang XC, Chung N, Gates A, Stec E, Kunapuli P, Holder DJ, Ferrer M, Espeseth AS (2006). "Robust statistical methods for hit selection in RNA interference high-throughput screening experiments". Pharmacogenomics **7** (3): 299–09. doi:10.2217/14622416.7.3.299

32. Brideau C, Gunter G, Pikounis B, Liaw A (2003). "Improved statistical methods for hit selection in high-throughput screening". Journal of Biomolecular Screening **8** (6): 634–47. doi:10.1177/1087057103258285. PMID 14711389

33. Cohen J (1994). "The Earth Is Round (P-Less-Than.05)". American Psychologist **49** (12): 997–1003. doi:10.1037/0003-066X.49.12.997. ISSN 0003-066X

34. Zhang XHD (2009). "A method for effectively comparing gene effects in multiple conditions in RNAi and expression-profiling research". Pharmacogenomics **10** (3): 345–58. doi:10.2217/14622416.10.3.345. PMID 20397965

35. Zhang XHD (2010). "Strictly standardized mean difference, standardized mean difference and classical t-test for the comparison of two groups". Statistics in Biopharmaceutical Research **2** (2): 292–99. doi:10.1198/sbr.2009.0074

36. Zhang XHD (2010). "Assessing the size of gene or RNAi effects in multifactor high-throughput experiments". Pharmacogenomics **11** (2): 199–213. doi:10.2217/PGS.09.136. PMID 20136359

37. Deprez-Poulain R, Deprez B (2004). "Facts, figures and trends in lead generation". Curr Top Med Chem **4** (6): 569–80. doi:10.2174/1568026043451168. PMID 14965294

38. Keserű GM, Makara GM (August 2006). "Hit discovery and hit-to-lead approaches". Drug Discov. Today **11** (15-16): 741–8. doi:10.1016/j.drudis.2006.06.016. PMID 16846802

39. Bleicher KH, Böhm HJ, Müller K, Alanine AI (May 2003). "Hit and lead generation: beyond high-throughput screening". Nat Rev Drug Discov **2** (5): 369–78. doi:10.1038/nrd1086. PMID 12750740

40. Cockbain J (2007). "Intellectual property rights and patents". In Triggle JB, Taylor DJ. Comprehensive Medicinal Chemistry **1** (2nd ed.). Amsterdam: Elsevier. pp. 779–815. doi:10.1016/B0-08-045044-X/00031-6. ISBN 978-0-08-045044-5.